MPRPM V2

MPRPM V2

Some days we all need a little more prayer. The human experience is ongoing, challenging, and downright scary. BUT, it is also beautiful, sacred, and everlasting. It's truly a glass half-full scenario! We may often see wicked individuals living a seemingly "free" life, causing harm onto others and chaos amidst God's realm. But always remember, their choices may allot instant "freedom" - (the same FREE WILL we all have), but theirs now has a physical expiration date. Don't let the wrongdoing of others discourage your course. The now is important, but the endgame is the key. The prayers inside are mostly focused on ourselves, as we are the main storyline. BUT, the prayers emphasize <u>we</u> being a better <u>me</u>! So, here's to you!

God Loves You. I Love You. We Love You.

To my Son,
You are truly a gift from God. My Heart, My Soul, My Mini. I Love You, boy.
MPRPM V2

1 - Dear Lord, I ask that You grant me the confidence necessary to believe in myself, as I believe in You. I ask for clarity as I traverse a convoluted reality. Allow me to walk in Your light, and see others as would You. Please help me stand confidently and move securely, as I attempt to provide the best of me to not just You, but to everybody. Help me capitalize on the strength You've blessed me with, and allow me to make the most of the gifts You've given. In Your Grace we pray, Amen.

2 – YHWH, I ask that You give special honor and appreciation to those that have guided me to You through dark times. Thank You for Your persistence; Your benevolence continues to shine as I receive Your word through the mouths of Your children, when needed the most. Please take some time today to bless those who righteously help others. May their hearts find the eternal peace and glory that You represent. Thank You for allowing such generosity to be carried from Soul to Soul, and Thank You for allowing mine to know growth. With Respect, Honor, and Love, I pray, Amen

3 – God, please help the lost souls stuck wandering our earth. There is pain, desperation, drug use, and maliciousness bastardizing the world today, using Your name in vain. I ask that, through Your Light, we can begin to repair the damaged souls and hearts that find themselves lost or Godless. Help those battling addiction, mental health, spirituality, and life. Please help those lost in the process of life to find Your light, and create structure in Your grace. In Your Glory I proclaim, Amen!

4 – Jesus, I pray that those struggling with addiction find Peace. May every kind, caring, and loving soul that battles the demons of addiction find an arsenal of tools available to their immediate use, ratifying the expungement of maliciousness. May they know, that, not only God loves them, but so do WE. May they know that they are not alone, and that there is a world without crippling pain, fear, and depression. Please help those understand that they are not alone, and that they are LOVED. In Your name I pray, Amen.

5 - Holy God, I call on the Legion of Angels, Helpers, and Souls of Your Light, utilized to spread the Word of YHWH. I ask that each and every Deity, Soul, and Angel tasked with His mission find the strength and ability to easily overcome any demon. I ask that we, as Your children, find safety in their presence and actions, and glorify their existence in the Light of Your Will. It is through You, in which all is possible. In Your presence we assemble, in Your name we pray, Amen.

6 - Our Father, please take the time today to bless my siblings. Throughout thick and thin, there is always someone I can count on. We may disagree, argue, spite and fight, but the love and bond remain, day and night. Please allow them to feel Your love, bless them with growth, and continue to steer them in Your direction, so that we may be the best versions of ourselves for one another and for You. Thank you for Your love, attention, time, and dedication. In Your name, God, we pray, Amen.

7 - Lord, help me with my sins. Allow me to cease committing those of which I know and educate me of those in which I am not yet aware of. Allow me to grow beyond my transgressions and point me to the inner strength You've provided, which is necessary to change my actions; creating a continuously improving me. Lord, I ask that You hear my true intentions and assist in diminishing my ego so that I may act in Your Will. Help me turn my sins into Holy actions, and my thoughts pure. With love and acceptance, Amen.

8 - Our Father, allot me growth and recognition, so that I may not take for granted all of which You have given. Allow me celebration and appreciation in moderation with all that You continue to provide. Let Your true Will apprehend my actions, and remind me to treat everyone with love, patience, and consideration. Lead me in my role of the unification of mankind, and may all of Your children find peace in Your intended world. I pray that everyone acts with a little bit more consideration to a neighbor or stranger alike. In Your peace, love, and will, Amen.

9 - Dear Jesus, Thank You for the sacrifices You made to allow me my daily breath. Thank You for sacrificing Your well-being, Your will, and Your flesh; allowing mankind the ability to continue the pursuit of life in the light of God's Love. Please help direct us back on Your intended path as a collected and unified people; allowing the world to heal. Please embrace all of those in the world facing oppression, hate, maliciousness, and deprivation. Protect us from such maliciousness. In Your grace we pray, Amen.

10 - Our Father, who Reign in Heaven, hallowed be thy name. Thy Kingdome come, Thy Will be done, on Earth as it is in Heaven. Give us this Day, our Daily Bread, and forgive us for our sins, as we forgive our sinners. Lead us not into temptation; but deliver us from evil. For thine is the Kingdom, the Power, and the Glory, as its been and as will be, Forever, Amen.

(Matthew 6:9-13 – The Lord's Prayer)

11 - Dear Lord, please help me act, think, and speak with patience. Allow me the emotional growth and maturity to NOT lash out at others. Allow me the growth and structure to NOT react when not necessary. Help me grow into the person You intend me to be! Please direct me towards the righteous path and steer me from the chaos surrounding. Lord, help my true intentions match Your true will. In Your grace we pray, Amen.

12 - God, allow me this day, this bread, and this water. Thank You for providing, endlessly, despite MY perception. Please help me create positivity, nourish growth, and demonstrate righteousness. Lead me to trust, as You trust me to lead. Help me to truly be a representation of God, day in and day out. In Your name we pray, Amen.

13 - Lord, bless the world. I pray for mother earth, that it may not be consumed by darkness. Your Will is foreign, but YOU are present. Despite the chaos, You remain unshaken; allotting guidance, peace, and love to those who seek it through You - You keep Your word. For this, I must Thank You for guiding me into the light and onto the path of which You intend. Allow me growth, wisdom, and determination. Amen.

14 - Lord, I pray for my parents. Bless those who raised me, and those who tried. Allow happiness, good health, and peace to frequent their days. May they find an abundance of Your comfort, embrace, and love. Thank You for placing them in my life and allowing us to learn from one another. In Your grace and Will we pray, Amen.

15 - Good Food, Good Meat, Great God! Let's Eat! Lord, Thank You for this bountiful meal. Bless all of those who contributed, and may this meal nourish our body, mind, spirit, and soul. Please allow those who may not be as fortunate to find sustenance and receive nourishment. May we all continue to eat well, without gluttony or sin. Thank You for all that You provide; from beginning to end, Amen.

16 – Dear Jesus, please protect us while we travel. As we embark on this journey, please shield us in Your White Light. Allot us protection from maliciousness and steer us from evil. Walk at our side as we traverse common and uncommon ground alike, and navigate us through uncertain waters. May we find adventure safely, and return home timely. With love and appreciation, we pray, Amen.

17 - Dear Lord, as the winds howl and the rain falls, I ask for Your protection. When the fire rages, and the water rises, we ask for Your mercy. Place a shield of Light surrounding us and our home. Enable Your energy and presence to surround us and shield us from any damage that may come forth. Please keep us safe! Alas, allow safety and protection for anyone within reach. In Your Power we praise, Amen!

18 - Dear Lord, we are in
need of assistance. We ask that
You visit _______, and restore their
inner-power and health. Allow
the positive energies of Your
creations to cleanse the ailment
from their body. We ask that You
remove the malicious energies
and spirits that may be attacking.
Remove illness, sickness, and
contagion. Help their body
restore itself and create a path for
recovery, as fit in Your Will.
Please embrace them as they
fight for wellness. In Your Grace,
Light, and Acceptance we pray,
Amen.

19 – God, grant me rest; grant my body power - grant my soul protection - grant my mind clarity. Please help me remove the ill-fated contaminants within my body. Allow me Samson strength, Your Holy breath, and the blessing of Jesus in knowledge. God it is through Your Will in which all is possible, and through Your intention in which all is procured. Deliver me from sickness, as You see fit, and provide me opportunity. Alas, God, I ask that You direct me to the medicine in which You intend for my healing or my comfort. In Your Wisdom and Guidance, I pray, Amen.

20 - Dear Lord, Guide _____ to Your Light. As You call them home, please embrace them. Steer them to Your Glory, and welcome them into Your domain. Comfort them as they sleep, and extend our appreciation for the moments we keep. Thank You for allowing _____ to bless my existence with laughter, love, and wisdom. Help me be the best I can be, not just for myself, but for them as well. With You, all is possible, and in Your name we pray, Amen.

21 - Dear God, please help me retain my confidence and trust in Your Will. Allow me to disperse of the animosity when failing to recognize Your plans. Help me improve my spiritual connection with You, and allow structure to overcome my faith, finding residence in my earthly existence. Thank You for continuously paving a path, and inspiring me to share humility, empathy, and consideration. Through You, all is possible, and with You, no evil shall prevail. In Your name we praise, Amen.

22 – El, Adonai, Elohim, The God of gods, and the King of kings, Thank You for allowance. Thank You for each and every blessing, each and every day. God, You continue to lead me through all of which I face, and You continue to provide love, confidence, and grace. You are the holiest of holies, yet You have the time and power to Love each of us as our own, for who You created us to be. God, continue to humble me, and continue to guide me. Through You, I can be of God, by Your design. With love, admiration, and respect, Amen.

23 - Dear God, I cannot begin to Thank You enough for my child(ren). They are everything You built in me, and everything I failed to be. You have allowed a new soul to grow and thrive in the Light of Your Love, and I am lucky enough to be their parent. Thank You for trusting me to raise them to Your intention, and please continue to guide me as necessary to ensure I parent in the Light of God, nurturing their soul to the Light of Your Will. I am humbly in awe, and forever in appreciation. In Your Love and Trust I give thanks, Amen.

24 – Dear Michael, Raphael, Gabriel, Uriel, Camael, Jophiel, and Zadkiel please allow and assist me to pray with Godly intention and with the utmost and necessary humanly-power. Help me stand without fear, sleep with peace, and act as God intends. Guide me as a Warrior of God, and allow me to prepare myself for my next chapter of God's plan. Thank You each for representing, protecting, and loving us. Thank You for Your sacrifices. In God's name we pray, Amen.

25 - Dear Lord, please help guide me through and to truth! Allow me to act in Your light and direct me to Your intended path. Allow me to act, and view with and in honesty, as You view Your children. Allow me to be as You see fit, and drive me to be better than I believe I can be. Thank You for Your trust, wisdom, and guidance. Through You, all is possible, and with You, no weapon formed against me shall prosper. In Your grace I worship, Amen.

26 - Lord! Thank You for the loving bundles of joy You have provided in the form of my pet(s). Your continuous Love, ceaseless forgiveness, and bountiful appreciation carries forward everyday within my faithful companion. Dear Lord I ask that You allow me to provide the best care possible for my friend and keep them close to Your heart so that they may continue to strengthen mine. Thank You, Lord. In Your Glorious name we praise, Amen!

27 – YHWH, glory and appreciation to You! Thank You for guiding me into and within my career. Please allow me to be the best of which I can be, and help me focus on the positive joys that my job has to offer. Please continue to open my heart and eyes to all of those around me, and assist me in being the best possible friend, mentor, co-worker, support, leader, and employee around. Through YOU, all is possible, and with You, all is able. I ask for Your continued guidance and discovery of my own strengths, so that I may act and walk in Your light, ceaselessly. God, in Your name we pray, Amen.

28 - Dear Lord, I find myself regularly asking for Your guidance and assistance. Though, I will always seek Your Light, I do ask for the personal strength to recognize my own ability in which You entrusted to me prior to birth. Lord, allow me to act in Your light, daily, as if I was receiving a non-stop stream of guidance. Help me continue to find the gifts You placed within my soul, and challenge me to be better, by no less than 1%, every day. Thank You for trusting me to act as a child of God, and continue pushing me when I need said encounter. In Your grace we give thanks and prayer, Amen.

29 - Lord, bless me with alignment. Allow my morals, goals, and ideals to be that of Yours. Please continue to drive me to and through Your path. Help me see all of life in which You've created. As I learn through You, I aspire to be of You. I genuinely appreciate the opportunities You continue to allot. As I grow and develop I pray to follow Your lead, and envelop my soul with Your direction, intention, and comprehension. Lastly, Lord, help me refrain from placing my earthly ideals of success over Your intentions for success. In Your Light I pray, Amen.

30 – Lord, please help me source viable food and drink to adequately nourish my body. Similarly, allow me the strength and help me build my discipline to consume what is necessary, not more, and what is righteous. Dispel the malicious energies that may have entered my body through excessively processed and modified foods. Thank You for providing sustenance and allow me to treat my body as You intended. In Your Love, Amen.

31 - Heavenly Father, Thank You for continuing to bless me with opportunities to share Your grace. As You continue to mold me into a Leader, allow me the patience and understanding to embrace the lessons You teach. Develop me and guide me to utilize the power You have placed within; to lead honestly, accurately, and wholly. Correct me always as I misstep! Thank You for trusting me to embrace and share in Your intention. With the upmost humility and appreciation, Amen.

32 – Our Father! Protect those who protect us! Please take the time today to give special embrace to all of the frontline, behind the scenes, fallen, and forgotten heroes that work in various aspects to protect Your herd. Deliver every one of Your children from evil, and bless each of those who assist in Your deliverance. Blessed be are those of Faith, and righteous are those who fight for Faith! With love, respect, and consideration for every Protector on earth, Amen!

33 – Dear Lord, please help bring home all Your children who have wandered astray. Help the hurt, the overly righteous, scared, and prideful. Help the lost, confused, and saddened souls that may have missed Your lessons on the ceaselessly yielding extent of Your welcoming. Please call all of those lost or looming close to Your presence, so that they can elect with their will, should it be, to walk home into the embrace and life intended by You, our Lord. Help those who are shameful, and fearful; help the addicted, conflicted, and unrestricted. In Your Love I proclaim, Amen!

I Want What God Wants for me.

Some people argue that following God's Will is not free will, but I'll argue that it is. I'm freely choosing to make his will mine.

Why?

Because his intentions for me have a much better track record than my own!

- I prayed for money; yet I was delivered a path to financial freedom
- I prayed for insurmountable strength; and I was delivered a copious amount of turmoil
- I prayed for patience; yet I was delivered a beautiful

child, of which time will
always seem insufficient
- I prayed for time, in which
he granted me deeper
appreciation
- I once prayed for death; in
which he gave me life
- I pray for resilience, and he
has made me a Leader

Sometimes, what you really need in life isn't what you end up praying for. However, as we each gain alignment with God's Will, our prayers and reality tend to intertwine.

As Daijh loves to say;

Don't confuse the Lord's tests with the devil's quests!

We are praying for _you_!

MPRPM V2